Dreams

How to Understand the Meanings and Messages of your Dreams. All about Lucid Dreaming, Recurring Dreams, Nightmares and more!

Felix M. White

Contents

Chapter 1. A Look at What Dreams Really Are.. 9

Chapter 2. How Dreaming Can Affect Emotional Stability..16

Chapter 3. How Dreams Help with Real Life Problems.. 24

Chapter 4. Dreaming & Your Stress Levels 33

Chapter 5. Dreaming to Help with Depression 41

Chapter 6. A Little about Lucid Dreaming & Its Benefits 49

Chapter 7. Dreams & How They Affect Your Memory..57

Chapter 8. How Dreams Help You to Become Self-Aware... 64

Chapter 9. A Few Ways to Avoid Nightmares & Keep Dreams Healthy 71

Chapter 10. A Few Things to Always Keep in Mind with Dreaming 79

© **Copyright 2019 by Felix M. White- All rights reserved.**

This document is geared toward providing exact and reliable information in regard to the topic and issue covered. The publication is sold with the idea that the publisher is not required to render accounting, officially permitted, or otherwise, qualified services. If advice is necessary, legal or professional, a practiced individual in the profession should be ordered.

- From a Declaration of Principles which was accepted and approved equally by a Committee of the American Bar Association and a Committee of Publishers and Associations.

In no way is it legal to reproduce, duplicate, or transmit any part of this document in either electronic means or in printed format. Recording of this publication is strictly prohibited and any storage of this document is not allowed unless with written permission from the publisher. All rights reserved.

The information provided herein is stated to be truthful and consistent, in that any liability, in terms of inattention or otherwise, by any usage or abuse of any policies, processes, or directions contained within is the solitary and utter responsibility of the recipient reader. Under no circumstances will any legal responsibility or blame be held against the publisher for any reparation, damages, or monetary loss due to the information herein, either directly or indirectly.

Respective authors own all copyrights not held by the publisher.

The information herein is offered for informational purposes solely, and is universal as so. The presentation of the information is without contract or any type of guarantee assurance.

The trademarks that are used are without any consent, and the publication of the trademark is without permission or backing by the trademark owner. All trademarks and brands within this book are for clarifying purposes only and are the owned by the owners themselves, not affiliated with this document.

Chapter 1. A Look at What Dreams Really Are

There are many beliefs on what dreams actually are, but dreams occur when we are unconscious and deep in sleep. A man named Sigmund Freud believed that they were windows into our unconscious. Dreams are images that our mind conjures while we are asleep, and they can include the five senses. You may still hear sounds, voices, have thoughts, and experience sensations while you're sleeping even though your physical body is laying there asleep. Often, a dream will have people you know in them, and you'll often see places that you've been. However, sometimes the mundane doesn't cut it and we'll dream of fantastical things, but we're pulling it from somewhere.

How do people accomplish the imagery needed for dreams and does it affect people physically?

Some people believe that we pull dreams for a collective unconscious, but it is generally believed that the images we see in dreams is something that we're subconsciously remembering from movies, posters, and things we catch sight of while we're awake in the physical world. Dreams hold our deepest fears and desires, and that's why sometimes you'll find that you dream of something you want to do. It's also why many people believe that they're a look into your unconscious mind or at least the subconscious mind.

Dreams can occur during almost any stage of sleep, but they are more abundant during the R.E.M. stage while you sleep. This is when they're easiest to remember. Your eyes are moving around during the R.E.M. cycle, rapidly beneath your eyelids. Your breathing is inconsistent, and your heart rate is also inconsistent. It's not as frightening as it sounds, but it is the only thing that keeps us from acting out dreams in the physical world. This makes dreaming safer.

So why do we dream? Does anyone know?

People know what dreams are, but people do not yet understand why we dream. There is a lot of speculation on the subject, but it is an indisputable fact that dreams help to benefit us mentally and emotionally. There are even some benefits that reach into the physical world.

Many people believe that dreams are directly related to our emotional stability because when people dream the limbic part of the brain is activated. The limbic part is the emotional part. Of course, the dorsal lateral prefrontal cortex is under-activated, which is more of the executive part. This leads people to believe that dreams are emotionally high, and that's what makes them so vivid, illogical, and often downright bizarre.

One of the benefits of understanding your dreams is emotional stability, and dreams are able to help guide you in your life. This is why this theory is known to make so much sense. In ancient times people thought that dreams were where people were able to receive wisdom given to them from the gods, and that is because dreams do provide you guidance in your life if you can discern what they mean. Of course, we know that dreams aren't a portal to another world, even though many still believe it is a portal to a spiritual plane that exists within our own world.

So do dreams really pose benefits? Should everyone dream?

Not everyone remembers their dreams, but everyone does experience them. You'll find that dreams do really pose many benefits that you can enjoy. Lucid dreaming is even something that you can experience to help you throughout your life as well. If you're dreaming, your stress is usually less, depression is fought off, it'll affect your physical comfort, and dreams can help you to solve problems. If you dream, it can actually help your memory as well. There are some practices you can use to make the process easier and ensure that you can remember what you see and experience at night.

Getting enough R.E.M. sleep will also help you to produce more proteins, which will help you to function better during the day. One way to increase your chances of remembering your dreams is to go to bed without too much stress on your mind, and meditation is usually best if you are having a hard time accomplishing this. Even simple breathing meditations can help you to relax your body and focus your mind, pushing negativity and stressors away from your conscious mind so that your subconscious can settle enough to allow for proper sleep.

If you are not reaching R.E.M. sleep, you're more likely to experience depression, anxiety, and overall negativity. People need dreams and the R.E.M. cycle to help be more positive when they wake up and feel well rested after a long night's sleep. It doesn't matter if you're sleeping eight hours because if you aren't hitting the

R.E.M. cycle, then you're not getting a restful night's sleep.

One way to ensure that you hit the R.E.M. cycle and experience more pleasant dreams is to stop being a night owl. If you're a night owl, you're actually more likely to have nightmares and have trouble hitting the R.E.M. cycle. Going to bed a little early makes the difference, allowing you to dream peacefully and reap the benefits of it.

Chapter 2. How Dreaming Can Affect Emotional Stability

Dreams can affect emotional stability, and if you want to function properly within society and be the best version of yourself that you can be, you need to be emotionally stable. It's more than just avoiding depression because dreams are able to help you to come to terms with grief, become more confident and assertive, and become emotionally whole. If you start lucid dreaming, then it is even more likely that you'll be able to balance your emotional state through your dreams, but dreams have an inherent effect on your emotional state even if you can't directly control them.

What is the importance of emotional stability?

There are many benefits to achieving emotional stability, and that is because having emotional stability will help you to be more confident in your everyday life. This will then help you to achieve your goals. You are more likely to be able to handle problems head on, and it'll help you to process negative emotions as they come along during the day.

Emotions have to be controlled if you want to be successful in life and not form negative habits. Emotional stability allows you to take criticism in a mature manner, act on your maturity, develop maturity, and keep from becoming too easily irritated or angry. It is also what allows you to accept negative people and situations.

Being able to control your emotions is what allows you to make judgment calls that won't come back to bite you later. It can help you in personal relationships, social situations, work, and even at school. It'll help you to reach goals by understanding how you should act during each situation that is thrown at you, and it'll make sure that you gain the maturity you need to keep moving forward in your life, both personal and goal related.

How do dreams help you to understand your emotions and gain emotional stability?

There are many different ways that dreams will help you with emotional stability, and one of the first ways is that dreams can help you to gain confidence. Confidence is important, and it is based on how you feel about yourself and your capabilities. Being able to recall your dreams will help you to become more assertive and more confident. Even if what happened in the dreamscape didn't happen in real life, you've gained some knowledge of how you'd react in a situation and what you feel that you can do. You reap this benefit by recalling those dreams, allowing you to be a more confident and assertive person. It's a way to confront and express your feelings, and that is one reason that it is recommended you write down your dreams if you are having a hard time remembering them. If you have written down the situations you've faced in your dreamscape and your reaction, then you'll be able to draw strength from those dreams, and your memory will be a little clearer.

Dreams also help you to confront your emotions head on, as dreaming is considered to be a very emotional aspect of your life because when you are dreaming it is the emotional part of your brain that is active. Everyone has stressful aspects present in their lives, and that means that you have negative emotions that may be weighing you down as well. Anger is one of the main emotions that dreams help you to face, and you can't deny your emotions in your dreams. The emotions that you experience while dreaming is involuntary. This means that you have to face them before you can move past them.

Can dreams help with more than just anger?

Yes, and you'll find that in your dreams you experience a full range of emotions from lust, fear, anger, general desire, happiness and every emotion in-between. All of your emotions need to be accepted and in balance if you want to gain emotional stability, and with dreaming you'll be forced to confront all of your emotions in the dreamscape. You can even overcome fears and phobias when it comes to dreaming, but this usually accomplished through lucid dreaming, which will be covered in a later chapter.

Everyone has a fear that they need to confront, and while you're awake, you're more likely to avoid these fears and phobias, denying that they are there, than when you're asleep. When you're asleep you have nowhere to go, and you'll have confront what is bothering you. This is the same for lust or other emotions. If you are having issues with an emotion that you are trying to stay in denial about, dreams will expose that emotion, making you confront them as soon as you wake up.

What is the best way to reach emotional stability through your dreams?

Other than lucid dreaming, if you want to reap the benefit of emotional stability from your dreaming experience, you'll need to write your dreams down and reflect on them. You'll gain some stability from just facing your emotions and coming out of denial, but true emotional stability comes from being able to face emotions, ask yourself why you're feeling these emotions, and consciously coming up with a solution to move past these emotions or how to accept them as a whole.

For example, if you are dreaming about a loved one and you are continuously arguing with them. Even if you're not arguing physically or verbally with them while you're awake, you're most likely mad at them. Otherwise, you would not be having these dreams about your loved one. If you feel you aren't angry with them, this is a part of the denial process. By remembering your dreams, writing them down, and reflecting on them, you'll be able to determine what you're mad at. Even if you never find out what you are mad at, by not denying the emotion that you are experiencing, you'd be able to move past it.

Without your dreams, this would not be possible because you would not have recognized that your subconscious was holding onto anger or a feeling of betrayal, causing the anger. Reflecting on your dreams and forcing yourself to realize any emotions you are trying to deny, will help you to gain the emotional stability and maturity that you need to handle everyday situations and meet your goals.

Chapter 3. How Dreams Help with Real Life Problems

Dreams can help with real life problems because they give you insight as to what's bothering you. All you have to do is learn how to interpret them. Dreams are an indication that you're not very balanced, and they help you to seek to become balanced.

It is important that you find your life to be meaningful, purposeful, and guided in some manner. Many people believe that dreams are the body's way of guiding you through the tough decisions you don't want to face in the waking world. Other people believe that dreams are guidance from a higher power. Either way, dreaming can help you to solve issues that you are facing and navigate the tough and confusing waters of the waking world.

How do you reap this benefit of dreaming?

If you want to reap this benefit, you need to learn to take action when you dream. Once you've had an insightful dream, and every dream can be considered insightful, you need to take action so that you can follow the guidance that was given to you. This also requires that you learn how to interpret your dreams correctly. Even simple things in your dreams can represent something great.

It's more than just knowing that a bird can symbolize freedom. Instead, some meanings are changed by the surrounding area in the dream, and you must learn to figure it out by asking yourself if these images have personal meaning as well. You cannot reap this benefit passively, and instead you have to work hard to discern and act on the messages given to you in your dreams.

How do you start the interpretation process?

Starting the interpretation process is as easy as telling someone your dream. Sometimes, you can just write it out. The words you use to describe a dream are extremely important in helping to discern the meaning of the elements in your dreams. You shouldn't worry about your dreams seeming disjointed because dreams aren't meant to follow a linear order.

Instead, your dreams are giving you the information that you need to act. You aren't given much more information than that. Of course, another reason that many people find their dreams to be too disjointed is that they are not used to remembering their dreams. You will remember the key elements, but small details may be lost until you practice remembering your dreams, which will increase your capacity to remember the details.

Once you write down your dreams, you'll start to remember more details. Over time, you'll remember all of the important details, and you'll be able to determine what your dreams are trying to tell you much easier. You'll need to write down what you think each element means, and you'll be able to create a meaning that once put into practice guides you.

What's an example?

Pretend you've dreamed the dream below:

I'm running through the forest. Then, suddenly I hit asphalt. There's nothing around me for miles. No people. I feel my heart pounding in my chest, and a sharp pain goes through my head. A single bird flies across the sky, but it's shot down from something I can't quite see. As the bird falls to the ground, I black out and wake up.

This is a relatively simple dream with a lot of elements in it. Now that the dream is written down, you can learn to interpret it by breaking the elements apart. Make a list of the elements and their possible meanings. For example:

- **Running in the forest:**
    - Running in a place you feel free
    - Running where your ancestors ran
- **Forest ending in asphalt:**
    - Ending in the modern world

- o Ending where nothing's natural
- **Nothingness:**
  - o A feeling of emptiness inside you
  - o A lack of meaning or definition
- **A feeling of pain and fear:**
  - o Feeling helpless
  - o Feeling ill
- **A bird flying:**
  - o Reaching out for freedom
  - o Trying to escape your surroundings
- **A bird being shot:**
  - o Being held down
  - o Unable to escape
- **Blacking out as it dies:**
  - o A connection to the bird
  - o A desire for freedom

You see that there are at least two possible meanings for each element. Now, you need to think about what makes sense to you. If you're connected to your ancestors, you're more likely to feel like that's what the dream is about. However, for most people it'll just be a place that's free and natural. Take that into consideration for the next aspect, and you'll find out that the meaning is nothing is natural around you.

That leads you to believe you lack meaning in your life because you feel like everything is fake, and that will lead to a feeling of helplessness. You can interpret the rest as trying to escape your surroundings but being held down by something despite your desire for freedom.

What do you do next? How do you apply it?

Now, once you've picked your interpretations. Apply it all together.

I feel trapped in a world where nothing is natural or real, and I've run into nothing but emptiness. There's no meaning. I feel helpless because I can't escape this place in my life, and something is holding me down. I can't reach freedom.

Now that you've figured out what your dream was trying to tell you, you can apply it to the world around you. Ask yourself why you feel that nothing is real and that the world is empty. Why are you feeling helpless? What do you think is holding you down? Was there a detail in your dream you were forgetting? Why can't you reach freedom?

With dream interpretations, you are guided to ask the questions you need to, and you'll then be able to find more details in the dream that will help you to answer these questions. For example, you can feel that your job is holding you down or the people that are around you. Either way, you now know that most of your frustration, anger, anxiety, fear and stress is stemming from that feeling of despair and lack of freedom. You've been guided to your problem, and when you act on the guidance you received, you'll be happier.

Chapter 4. Dreaming & Your Stress Levels

Stress is a negative factor in your life that can stop you from achieving your goals, drop your immune system, and has negative effects on your life overall. Dreams are also known to help relieve stress from emotional pain. People who are stressed have difficulty sleeping in the first place, and that creates a negative cycle because lack of sleep can cause stress on its own. You have to break this cycle if you want to reap this dreaming benefit.

How do dreams help you to relieve stress?

Sleep is extremely fundamental to your health, and a sign of healthy sleeping is healthy dreaming. This is why you need to dream to be a more balanced person. Not to mention that sleeping helps you to gain self-awareness, which is also going to lower your stress. Many of the overall benefits that you achieve from sleep will also help you to relieve stress over time.

This is why it is so important to build healthy patterns of sleep. Dreams are a type of therapy that you can achieve overnight, and this is because of neurochemical composition that is found in the dream state of our sleep. It helps to remove the edges of emotional stressors, and it acts like a soothing balm applied to emotional wounds that have accumulated throughout the day.

When you hit the R.E.M. stage of sleep, your norepinephrine, which is a chemical that is produced by the brain and associated with stress, decreases. During the dreaming process, you are reprocessing the events of that day, even if you aren't reliving them directly. This softens the emotional impact of those experiences, which decreases the amount of stress that you feel from the previous day. It will help you to cope with bad experiences and feel refreshed and ready to take on anything, both the good and bad, which a new day has to offer.

Without sleep, you will not experience this drop in norepinephrine, and your stress is more likely to just pile up, making it harder to function in the days to come. This can lead to anxiety and depression disorders. It can cause your sleep to become disrupted as well, which can lead to a variety of health conditions. To relieve stress properly throughout the night, you need to enter R.E.M. and experience healthy dreams, which will allow you to work through your stressors and your overall problems.

How do you have healthy dreams if you're already stressed?

To have healthy dreams if you are already stressed you are going to need to break the cycle. This is easier said than done, but it's a needed step to experiencing a more positive sleeping experience that will help you to decrease your stress levels as a whole and cope with negative feelings and experiences. There are many ways that you can go about breaking the cycle, and some ways will work better for certain people than others.

Starting a healthy sleep routine is usually the best way to break the habit. The first way to decrease your stress through dreams is being able to enter the dreaming cycle with ease and while you're in a positive mindset. Some people find that it is easier to mediate or drink tea, but there are also alternatives to this. You can listen to soothing sounds or music before bed, and this will put many people in the right state of mind.

Always make sure that you're relaxed before bed. If you're tense, you're more likely to be irritated as you go to sleep, and you're more likely to have nightmares or not be able to dream because of it. This will worsen your stress instead of relieving it. If you are having trouble sleeping because of something in your environment, such as a bad bed, it is important that you replace that bed to improve your quality of sleep. This in turn will improve your quality of dreams. Another stressor in your environment which can cause you to have interrupted sleep and difficulty dreaming or remembering your dreams is exposure to light.

If you are on an odd sleep schedule, it is recommended to invest in black out curtains to help keep out the light. If you are having issues with lights that are already present in your room, then you can invest in a sleeping mask to help you block out this light as well. You can even get a soothing sleeping mask that is padded with cooling gel or lavender scented to help you relax. Getting to sleep with a positive attitude and sleeping restfully is key to breaking the negative cycle.

Can dreams help you to recognize stress so you can consciously decrease it?

Yes, dreams can also help you to recognize your stress, and this will help you to consciously work on decreasing your stress. Of course, to reap this benefit, you have to understand how to interpret dreams and find what is really stressing you out, even when the dream appears to be nonsensical.

There are times that dreaming is easier to interpret than others, and if you are having a vivid dream that follows a logical sequence of events, then you're more likely to be able to work on a problem that is bothering you. Once you either accept the problem or find a solution for it, sometimes both, you'll be able to cut that stress out of your life or at least decrease it.

However, even if your dreams aren't following a rational line of events, it is still possible to figure out what is stressing you. Your dreams build connections from what is stressing you to something that can also be put into that category or represent the problem. By learning to interpret your dreams, you'll be able to figure out the problem and then find a solution no matter how nonsensical your dream is. No matter what, it will usually help to write your dreams down. This will help to make sure that you do not miss important details that may help you to relieve your stress levels later on.

Chapter 5. Dreaming to Help with Depression

Many people deal with depression, and it's a hard illness to get rid of. Depression is a mental illness that can affect you mentally, emotionally and even physically. Commonly, you'll notice a lowered immune system and weight gain when you are depressed. It is important to overcome depression, and you can do so naturally if you are experiencing healthy sleep and dream cycles. With depression it is important to stimulate positive dreams and minimize nightmares, even when they are naturally occurring.

How do dreams affect depression?

You may be wondering what the correlation between dreams and depression is, but the fact is that your depression can be caused or worsened by not getting enough sleep. When you are dreaming happy and vivid dreams, then you are sleeping well at night, which is going to help you get out of your depression or stave off depression all together.

If you are having bad dreams, you are most likely experiencing stress, anger, and anxiety. These are linked to depression, and negative emotions will convert into negative energy even in the waking world. It shows up as stress and irritation at first, but it builds and turns into full on depression, which is hard to get rid of.

Dreams are not depressed by nature, but it is easy to get lost in depressing dreams if you are not controlling your stress levels. If you are a lucid dreamer, it is easier to face your depression head on. When you are not in control of your dreams, it is harder to turn them towards a positive manner if you're in a rut of negativity. However, it is extremely important that you turn your dreams into a healthy direction if you want to be able to fight off or defeat the depression that you are experiencing.

So why do healthy dreams help to combat depression?

Healthy dreams will help you to combat depression because they are related to emotional stability, as explained in a previous chapter. You will also experience happier emotions when you are experiencing healthier dreams. This will mean that you'll be able to experience confidence, assertiveness, happiness, love, and even lust. These can be beneficial at counteracting the negativity that we face in the waking world or in our previous dreams. It'll help you to relieve stress, and by building your confidence and waking refreshed, you'll be ready to tackle the day and everything that it has to offer, both the good and the bad.

Dreaming can be a direct reflection of what we want out of life, and therefore it can help you to keep your goals in mind. When you achieve your goals in your dreams, you are more likely to feel like you can achieve them in the physical world when you're awake as well. Motivation is half the battle if you want to be successful, and with a successful night of rest and dreaming, you'll be more motivated to start your day.

After a pleasant dream, you'll also be starting the day on a good foot, which will help you to stay more positive during the day. This is important if you are trying to fight or keep depression away. Depression doesn't happen over just one bad day, but if you continuously start the day on a bad foot, then you are setting yourself up to experience depression.

What are a few things that you can do to help promote healthy dreams?

Remember that getting to sleep is the first step to enjoying your dreams, whether you're a lucid dreamer or not. This means that you should go to sleep relaxed, and many people will mediate or have a cup of relaxing tea before bed. Lavender or chamomile tea usually work the best, but remember to sweeten it with something natural like honey instead of sugar. Too much sugar is known to cause nightmares as well, so it'd be counterproductive to sweeten a bedtime tea with sugar, artificial or not.

Another way to help you promote good dreams is to make sure you are completely relaxed before going to bed. Sometimes this means that you should tire yourself out in a healthy way, and exercising after dinner is a good way to do that. This is also the reason that you shouldn't have caffeine right before going to bed. If you are too hyper to get to sleep, your dream cycle will be interrupted, and you'll get a poor night's sleep. This can further depression instead of stopping it.

Having a regular routine is also going to help you to get to sleep faster and a little more effectively. If you want to have a healthy R.E.M. cycle that leads to positive dreams, go to bed thinking positive thoughts. Many people will mediate before bed, but you can add in a positive mantra as well. Reassure yourself of your confidence and self-worth before bed, it'll go a long ways to promoting healthy dreams and keeping depression at bay.

If you are a lucid dreamer are you less likely to experience depression?

Everyone is able to experience depression, and it has more to do with how you experience life while you're awake that will cause depression. However, if you are lucid dreamer, you are more likely better able to combat negativity during the waking world by creating a dreamscape that makes you feel free and happy.

For example, many lucid dreamers experience a sense of freedom through their dreams, including the abilities they have in them such as flying. This is something that a normal dreamer will not be able to experience, and it is harder for a normal dreamer to combat depression because they cannot create a happy environment in their dreams that will lighten their mood as much as those who can dream lucidly. If you are battling depression, learning lucid dreaming can be extremely beneficial at helping you to fight it.

Chapter 6. A Little about Lucid Dreaming & Its Benefits

You may be wondering what lucid dreaming actually is, and in short is the ability to control your dreams. It can lead many people to experience an out of body experience or astral projection, but lucid dreaming is much more commonly the ability to control and shape your dreamscape. There are many benefits to lucid dreaming, and there are many ways to gain the ability to lucidly dream. Lucid dreams are often more vivid and easy to remember. There are many more benefits to lucid dreaming than just regular dreaming, and it'll help you to reap even more benefits from the time you spend asleep.

So what are the benefits of lucid dreaming?

You're likely to be more positive if you are able to lucidly dream, and that's because you can experience a confidence boost from being able to control your dreams. It'll allow you to become the hero and interact with anything or anyone that you want. This often allows you to be more assertive in the waking world as well. You can experience more when you're lucidly dreaming, and it tends to make people more adventurous when they're awake as well by removing the fear of the unexpected.

Many lucid dreamers will discover more meaning to life as well, and usually it's a personal meaning that will help them to get through even the toughest situations. People who can control their dreams usually believe that they have more control in the waking world as well, and they understand that they may never know the true meaning to life. Instead, they find comfort in the fact that they can create a meaning if nothing else, just like they do in their dreamscapes. This comfort that is gained from lucid dreaming has a far reaching effect on your outlook on life, helping you to stay motivated and face hard situations head first.

You're more likely to gain self-awareness from your dreams if you are lucidly dreaming as well. This is because in your lucid dream you can pull up yourself and have a conversation with different parts of who you are. It'll help you to observe your actions and face facets of your personality that you may be trying to deny. It is important that you never deny who you are or what you want if you want to be happy in life.

If you're having a hard time with fears and phobias, you may need more than an involuntary nightmare to help you get past it. That's why creating a lucid dream that helps you to face your fears safely is a great way to get rid of these fears and phobias. You know that you have control, and it helps you to realize that you can be in control of your actions and emotions. This will also transfer to more confidence in the waking world, and with less fears and phobias you have less holding you back from reaching your goals.

Getting over negative emotions and grief is also easier if you are able to lucidly dream, and that's because you'll be able to unite with loved ones. You'll even be able to yell at versions of your loved ones or friends so that you can get something off of your chest, which you can later do in real life if they are still around. When someone is gone and you never received closure, you can receive it in a lucid dream. This will help you to let go, and many people believe that lucid dreaming happens on the spiritual plane, so it is greatly debated on if you are truly able to talk to your loved ones one last time.

What else can lucid dreaming do?

One of the most important things that lucid dreaming can do for you is help you to realize your creative potential. Everyone has potential, and you have to recognize it if you want to be able to act on it. This acts as a motivation in the waking world, giving you the drive that you need to help reach all of your goals. You can push your limits and discover what you truly want in lucid dreams, and there is no one around to judge you but yourself.

How do you start lucidly dreaming?

There are many ways that you can start the journey to lucid dreaming, but one of the easiest ways is to start by just making sure you keep track of your regular dreams. This will help to increase your memory in relation to dreams, which opens the door to lucid dreaming later. Keeping a journal is usually recommended to help speed along the process.

Next, you're going to want to pick out dream signs as well. You need to find something in your normal dreams that will help you to know you're dreaming. Look for small inconsistencies, which many people will find once they start to write down their dreams.

These will be the cues you need to help wake you up in your dreams later.

It is also important that you take note of the waking world around you. You are conscious when you're wake, but you need to be focused as well. Think about everything you do, and it'll help you to control your dream body a little better. Focus on what it feels like to walk, and you'll be more likely to be able to move your muscles voluntarily in your dreams.

Keep asking yourself if you're dreaming, and the answer will obviously be no. However, you need to make sure that you understand why you're not dreaming. For example, if you were dreaming you could actually do anything you wanted. You would be able to defy gravity, for example. You'll remember this in your dreams.

After you've done this for a few days to a few weeks, you'll be able to start lucidly dreaming. The time varies on the person and how much effort you put into it. Wakeup in your dreams using the cues that you've picked out, and the simplest way is to recognize and repeat that you are dreaming. Then, the difficulty of staying lucid comes into play. Calm yourself down, or you'll wake yourself up. You'll learn to control your dreamscape from here, and sometimes small changes are easiest, and you'll need to practice like you would any other skill.

Chapter 7. Dreams & How They Affect Your Memory

Dreams are important if you want to have a sharp and focused memory, as dreaming is a sign that you are getting restful sleep and successfully entering the R.E.M. cycle. In your dreams you are already remembering things that even your conscious mind may not. Your dreams are a gateway to what you're feeling, what's bothering you, what you've seen that scares you, and everything that you see is pulled from somewhere.

It is believed that what you are seeing is pulled from the world that you've seen while awake even if you don't remember everything when conscious. For example, every face you see in your dreams is pulled from somewhere, but you may not remember every face that you've ever seen while awake. Dreams tie into your memory more than just remembering while you're dreaming though. If you are experiencing a healthy dream cycle, you're more likely to have a focused mind and better memory when awake.

So how do dreams really affect your focus and memory?

Your memory is important to your capacity to learn, and your dreams are known to help you with your memory. They are an extension of your learning capabilities. When you dream you are going to remember details of your memories, and one reason is because the level of cortisol, which is a stress hormone, will rise through the night. It will hit its peak while you're experiencing the R.E.M. period of your sleep.

This is supposed to help you work during your sleep, and that means that new experiences are going to be linked with old memories, strengthening that link so that you remember pieces of your old memories. This will later transfer into the waking world, and it'll help you to recall these old memories because you've developed more triggers to help you recall them.

Your brain works hard to solve issues in your life, including if you are frustrated over memory loss or trying to learn something new. Your brain will continue to work on these problems while you're asleep. This is why after a night's sleep you're more likely to be able to work out difficult problems, and your dreams will bring up older memories that are associated with what you're trying to learn. Once again, more triggers are being formed to strengthen your memory overall, allowing you to recall various facts and events.

Why is it important to strengthen your memory?

Your learning capabilities are increased when your memory is increased. People also tend to be happier if they are not having issues with their memory. If you are having issues remembering something that you feel is important, you feel less confident about yourself and your capabilities. This will lead to stress, and it can even lead to depression if you aren't careful. Strengthening your memory will help you to appear smarter because you are able to learn at a quicker rate, and it'll help you to improve on previous skills by being able to recall more that you learned and experienced on the subject. Intelligence is generally based on memory since it is what allows you to learn.

It will also help you to strengthen personal relationships because you'll learn how to recognize patterns if you can remember seeing them. This includes patterns in negative and positive behaviors, allowing you to navigate social events and relationships much more easily. By being able to remember what leads to positive reactions, you are able to create more positive reactions and events in your own life. This will improve your quality of life.

Can you get this benefit if you aren't sleeping well?

No, you won't be able to reap this benefit during the night if you aren't sleeping well in the first place. This is one of the main reasons that it is important that you minimize the amount of nightmares that you are having. It is also important that you strengthen your ability to remember your dreams as a whole.

If you remember your dreams a little better, you are going to remember the triggers that you've laid down to help you remember older memories better as well. So make sure to start with a dream journal and set yourself up for a good night's sleep so that you reap the full benefits that dreaming has to offer.

How can you increase your likelihood of improving your memory through dreams further?

To improve your memory through your dreams further, you can go to bed with a clear goal in mind. If you are a lucid dreamer, this is that much easier because you can create a dreamscape around what you're trying to remember. This is why lucid dreamers are known to be able to learn and enhance real life skills through their dreams, which is yet another reason to learn lucid dreaming. With lucid dreaming, you'll be able to practice for what seems like longer periods of time because everyone that remembers their dreams knows that it can feel like days even if only a few hours have really passed in the physical world.

Of course, you'll find that even if you aren't a lucid dreamer, if you go to bed with something clearly in your mind and without distraction, you are more likely to see it in your dreamscape. Even if it is not obviously present, your brain will be working on ways to set down triggers for the knowledge that you've learned so long as you've deemed it important.

Chapter 8. How Dreams Help You to Become Self-Aware

One of the main benefits of dreams is that you'll become more self-aware which is needed if you want to live a healthy and happy life. Many people do not know themselves, even if they think they do. This is why you are sometimes confused by your own actions, and it's important that you learn who you are and why you act the way you do. You are able to experience yourself as an individual if you know who you are, allowing you to think more independently. This will help to motivate you to make changes and strengthen your weaknesses so that you are a stronger person, becoming the best person you can be.

What are some benefits of self-awareness?

It may seem obvious, but one of the best parts of being self-aware is that you can understand and control your own emotions a little better. Emotional stability, as discussed before, is important in reacting in a positive manner even in a negative situation. It means that you're more likely to make good judgment calls if you are not confused by your own actions. For example, if you know yourself, then you know that you get angry when someone continuously says something or repeats a certain habit.

You will also become more confident if you are self-aware. This is because you know how you'll react, and you'll be able to direct your actions in a more positive manner. You'll also become more motivated, helping you to make sure that you push yourself in a positive manner. This will help you to set and obtain your goals.

You'll also be able to become more empathetic if you're self-aware. This is because when you understand your emotions a little better, you'll be able to understand the emotions and motivations of others. By knowing how people act, you'll be able to see patterns in how they react. This will help you to navigate social waters a little easier, acting more positively in social situations.

How do dreams help with self-awareness?

Dreams help you to become self-aware by making sure you can't deny how you feel. You can't hide who you are or what you feel in your dreams, and in one way or another it'll come up. Dreams will also help to tell your strengths and weaknesses. They reveal your fears, such as any phobia or fear you may be trying to suppress. With dreams, you'll also be able to tell what's stressing you, if something is stressing you, if you're not as confident as you thought you were, and so on.

You have to overcome any fear or doubt that you may have if you want to move forward in life. You have to be able to set goals, but you also need to be able to achieve those goals. This means that nothing should be holding you back, not even subconsciously. This is, once again, where writing and interpreting your dreams comes in handy. You'll be able to determine more about yourself.

With self-awareness, you'll be able to exhibit more leadership qualities, which will help you to get further in life. Dreams are good for more than just problem solving. Look for patterns in your dreams, and try to see if those patterns are also present in the waking world. Recognizing these patterns will help you to change them if necessary.

Such as if you feel down, you may go to alcohol in the waking world. This can lead to your dreams having you drowning in liquid, in a bar, or anything that may represent or revolve around alcohol. This will help you to become more aware of the vice that you're relying on, and it'll tell you that the vice is a negative habit. Now that you're self-aware of a bad coping mechanism, you'll be able to force a change in your life.

Do lucid dreamers have an advantage in achieving this benefit?

In a way, yes. Lucid dreamers are able to directly converse with their inner self if they choose to do so. They have to think about pulling their inner selves out of their subconscious mind, but by directly conversing with themselves they can get better insight on who they are or what they're trying to hide.

However, unlike normal dreamers, lucid dreamers have to ask the questions. Knowing what to ask is sometimes difficult on its own. They can ask to be shown something important, as they can give themselves guidance in this way. They can show you how to build confidence, what you're doing wrong, or you can just talk to yourself about how to solve a problem that is plaguing you.

In your dreams, you have more time to figure out what is bothering you and how to get past it. This is because while you're asleep and in a dream state, time seems to move differently than it does in the waking world. This makes it seem like you have more time than you're actually experiencing. One lucid dreaming session with yourself is more likely to give you results than hours of sitting there in the waking world and trying to figure out what a solution to your problem is.

If you're using this method to gain self-awareness, remember that your lucid dream self may not look like you. It can look like whatever you want it to be, and many people have a spirit side of them in their lucid dreams that seems to be more of a guiding spirit or even a spirit animal. However, this is your lucid dream self, and conversing with it will allow you to gain insight as to who you are and the best way for you to handle problems.

Chapter 9. A Few Ways to Avoid Nightmares & Keep Dreams Healthy

If you're trying to reap the benefits that good dreams and restful R.E.M. sleep has to offer, then it is important that you avoid nightmares as much as possible. Nightmares are bound to happen because they're only natural, but there are ways to minimize them as well. You don't always have to face your fears, except for when you're lucid dreaming and choosing to do so. Many nightmares are nonsensical as well, and if you cannot make sense of a nightmare, it is best to avoid it in the first place.

So what causes nightmares?

If you want to know how to avoid nightmares, you need to know a few causes of nightmares. Anxiety and stress is one of the main causes of nightmares. If you are going through a traumatic even or just an emotional one, you are more likely to have nightmares. Grief can also cause nightmares, or if you've witnessed a crime. It doesn't even have to be a grand tragedy to cause nightmares, as everyday stressors are known to cause nightmares as well, such as financial worries.

Another common trigger for nightmares is spicy food. This is because what you eat effects how you sleep. You'll spend more time awake after eating spicy food because of the digestive process and how harshly it affects it. This will cause bad dreams due to the disruption in your sleep patterns. For the same reason, you shouldn't eat too close to when you go to bed, even if you're eating non-spicy food. When you eat it'll increase your metabolism, and it'll also increase your brain activity, which prompts nightmares.

Alcohol is also known to cause bad dreams because it is a depressant. It'll help you to fall asleep, but as the alcoholic affects wear off you are going to wake up prematurely, setting yourself up for a bad night. If you consume alcohol too much, you're more likely to sleep poorly and go through alcohol withdrawal which will also cause nightmares.

Illness is also known to cause nightmares. This is mostly found in cases of the fever, such as when you have a cold or flu. The higher temperature will cause you to have nightmares, but sleep apnea can also cause bad dreams to occur.

Drugs that you may be on, prescribed or not, can cause nightmares as well. Narcotics, barbiturates and even antidepressants are known to cause nightmares as a side effect. If you already have bad dreams, then this can make it worse.

Fat content can also cause bad dreams, and that is why you shouldn't consume fatty foods during the day. Never consume fatty foods right before bed, but even consuming them during the day can be an issue. Junk food is just bad for your quality of sleep.

So what do you do to avoid nightmares?

When you are trying to avoid nightmares you need to avoid stressors. A healthy diet and exercise is going to help you sleep better, and it'll automatically help you to avoid fatty foods that will cause nightmares. You also should try to stay away from spicy foods, and make sure that you talk to your doctor if you are taking drugs that may cause you to have increased nightmares. Let your doctor know if you are experiencing these side effects right away.

When you are ill, try to lower your fever at least before you sleep. This way you are less likely to have fever dreams, which are a form of nightmares that are extremely emotional and yet very irrational. Never use alcohol to try and sleep if you are already experiencing nightmares, and it's not a good vice to have even if you aren't having nightmares, as it can cause them.

When you're already stressed or anxious about something, you'll want to try to lower your stress levels before you go to sleep to avoid nightmares and get the most out of your dreams and entering the R.E.M. cycle. There are many ways to lower your stress levels, and meditation is recommended to help with stress. It is a great way to center yourself, including mindfulness of breathing mediation, which will make you concentrate internally and finding balance and peace while concentrating on a physical sensation to distract you.

What are the benefits of avoiding nightmares?

Even though nightmares are natural, it is important that you limit the amount of nightmares that you are having so that they do not become a problem. Nightmares disrupt your sleep, leaving you open to depression, illness, affect your memory, increase your stress levels, and it can even lead to failure in meeting your goals. This is because if you are tired you are more likely to be irritated, irrational, and less motivated to push yourself.

Dreams have many benefits, including helping you to face real life problems once you interpret them. With nightmares, you won't find the same benefits as healthy dreaming and a restful night as well as an R.E.M. cycle. This is why you need to make sure to lower your risk of nightmares, but when you do experience the occasional nightmare, remember to face it head-on.

What do you do when you have a nightmare?

You'll need to accept that you had a nightmare, and if it doesn't repeat itself, then it's normal to have them. There may be something stressing you out in your life, so try to interpret the nightmare like you would for any other dream. This will help you to determine what you're having issues with in the waking world. If you're able to understand why you're having a nightmare, then you'll be able to fix the problem or at least start finding a solution to what is bothering you. Remember to reflect on your nightmares, denying them is more likely to cause them to repeat themselves and grow in intensity.

Chapter 10. A Few Things to Always Keep in Mind with Dreaming

One of the hardest parts about reaping benefits from healthy and happy dreams is making sure to ensure that you have healthy and happy dreams in the first place. This chapter is dedicated to tips and tricks to get better dreams and sleep well throughout the night. With these tips and tricks, you're more likely to reap the benefits that healthy dreams have to offer, and you'll feel more refreshed and ready to tackle anything that the waking world has to offer.

A Vitamin B6 Supplement:

Many people don't know that a vitamin B6 supplement is known to help with normal sleep function. You can add a supplement that's 100mg a day, and this will help you to increase the vividness that you experience in your dreams. It also increases the lucidness. Of course, before you take this supplement, you need to talk to a medical professional to see if it's safe to add into your normal daily routine. This is because it is above the recommended daily intake of vitamin B6, and you should always check to see if it's safe to add. Even if you only take the recommended dosage by your doctor, vitamin B6 is sure to help you make your dreams a littler clearer.

Use Foods to Help:

You already know that you shouldn't eat foods that are high in fat content or spicy before you to bed, as this can affect your dreams negatively. However, there are foods that will help to make your dreams a little more positive and vivid. You can eat foods that are high in vitamin B6, but you also want to eat foods that are high in tryptophan. Tryptophan helps you to treat depression, anxiety, regulate your sleep, and even helps to regulate your mood.

This can help increase the vividness of your dreams in a positive way. Sadly, you can't get a tryptophan supplement unless it's in the form of a prescription from your doctor. This is why consuming foods that are high in tryptophan is important. These are foods like turkey, tuna, venison, lamb, shrimp, cod, and even chicken. If you are looking for more vegetarian options tofu, pumpkin seeds and kidney beans are relatively high, but not as high as other meat options.

You have to consume these foods on a daily basis to really see any effect at all. That's because none of these foods have enough to make a difference after just consuming them once. However, adding it into your normal diet is a healthy dietary change that will help you to reap the benefits that your dreams have to offer.

Make Sure the Temperature is Comfortable:

It is important that the temperature in your room is comfortable if you want to sleep without interruption. If your sleeping environment is too hot or too cold, then your sleep is going to be disrupted, and you'll toss and turn most of the night instead of getting the sleep you need. This can stop you from entering the R.E.M. cycle, and it can disrupt your ability to remember or experience your dreams as a whole. This will stop you from reaping the benefits of your dream cycles dead in your tracks.

Think about Something Relaxing:

Even if your day was extremely stressful, you need to let it go before you sleep. This is the same reason that people should never go to bed mad. If you go to bed mad or stressed out, you are more likely to create nightmares. If meditation isn't for you, you need to make sure you have some method of letting go of stress. Sometimes, people will repeat a mantra again and again before bed.

This is usually an affirmation that you are confident, relaxed, or something else that gives you confidence. Do not repeat the mantra out loud, as this may keep you awake. However, saying it in your head is a great way to make sure that you're falling asleep with positive thoughts in your head, allowing you to get better rest and experience more pleasant dreams.

Put a Damp Cloth Over Your Eyes:

This may seem silly, but it really works. Your eyes can become tense throughout the day, and this will also keep you from resting well and reaching your dream cycle. Putting a slightly damp and cool cloth over your eyes helps your eyes to relax, which will help you to get to sleep faster. When you experience relief from the tenseness in your eyes, you will also experience less headaches and tension in the overall region. This is will reduce the likelihood of experiencing nightmares as well.

Create an Actual Schedule:

It's not enough to create a sleep schedule, but it is also important that you actually follow it. If you're just sleeping whenever you're tired, you're less likely to be sleeping properly. This will stop you from having healthy dreams and feeling rested when you get up. Despite being an adult, setting a bedtime is actually a necessary habit to have. You will also want to set an alarm so that you wake up in the morning around the same time every day. For a few days, it may seem tiresome as you get used to the schedule. However, after a while, you'll find that your body feels more rested and refreshed from following it.

Make sure that you're open to the idea that dreams can benefit you, and if you are open to understanding and following your dreams, you are much more likely to be able to use them to your advantage during your time awake. Stay calm, and never get frustrated because you don't understand a dream, and you're more likely to receive the guidance that you need to improve your life. Dreams will also help to stabilize your emotional and mental state, which is important if you are trying to live a healthy life. Through dreaming, you can learn to be more positive, find guidance, relive stress, fight off depression, and become a happier and healthier you.

www.ingramcontent.com/pod-product-compliance
Lightning Source LLC
Chambersburg PA
CBHW050203130526
44591CB00034B/2069